THE OSTEOPOROSIS EXERCISE BOOK

A Safe and Effective Program to Build Strong Bones

TABLE OF CONTENTS

INTRODUCTION

Osteoporosis is a common bone disorder characterized by the gradual weakening of bone density and quality, leading to bones becoming fragile and susceptible to fractures. It is often referred to as the "silent disease" because it typically progresses without noticeable symptoms until a fracture occurs. Osteoporosis can affect people of all ages and genders but is more common in postmenopausal women and older adults.

The condition occurs when the rate of bone resorption (the breakdown of old bone tissue) outpaces the rate of bone formation, resulting in a net loss of bone mass. Factors contributing to osteoporosis include hormonal changes, genetics, inadequate nutrition, sedentary lifestyles, and certain medications. Common risk factors include a family history of osteoporosis, low body weight, smoking, excessive alcohol consumption, and a lack of weight-bearing exercise.

The consequences of osteoporosis can be severe, with fractures occurring most commonly in the hip, spine, and wrist. These fractures can lead to pain, disability, loss of independence, and even a reduced life expectancy, particularly in the case of hip fractures.

Exercise plays a crucial role in the management and prevention of osteoporosis. It helps improve bone density, balance, strength, and overall physical function. However, not all exercises are suitable for individuals with osteoporosis, and safety precautions must be observed. Weight-bearing exercises are essential for improving bone density. These activities involve supporting your body's weight through your bones and muscles. Examples include walking, jogging, hiking, dancing, stair climbing, and low-impact aerobics.

Strength training, also known as resistance or weight-bearing exercise, helps build and maintain muscle mass, which, in turn, supports and strengthens bones. Focus on exercises that target the major muscle groups, such as squats, lunges, leg presses, and bicep curls. Balance and posture exercises help reduce the risk of falls and fractures. These exercises improve stability and coordination, crucial for individuals with osteoporosis. Yoga, tai chi, and specific balance drills are beneficial. Stretching exercises enhance joint mobility and flexibility. Activities like gentle yoga or daily stretching routines can help improve overall flexibility and reduce the risk of injury from falls.

Low-impact activities like swimming, water aerobics, stationary cycling, and elliptical training provide cardiovascular benefits without placing excessive stress on the joints, making them suitable for individuals with osteoporosis. Strengthening the core and back muscles can improve posture and reduce the risk of spine-related fractures. Exercises such as planks, bridges, and back extensions are effective. Deep breathing exercises and relaxation techniques can help reduce stress and promote relaxation, which is essential for overall well-being.

It's important to consult with a healthcare provider or a physical therapist before starting any exercise program, especially if you have osteoporosis or other underlying health conditions. They can assess your individual condition, provide tailored exercise recommendations, and ensure that you exercise safely and effectively. Additionally, gradually progress your exercise routine and listen to your body to prevent overexertion and minimize the risk of injury. Exercise, when done correctly and under professional guidance, can be a powerful tool in managing and preventing osteoporosis.

PART ONE

WHAT IS OSTEOPOROSIS?

Osteoporosis is a disease that weakens your bones. It makes your bones thinner and less dense than they should be. People with osteoporosis are much more likely to experience broken bones (bone fractures). Your bones are usually dense and strong enough to support your weight and absorb most kinds of impacts. As you age, your bones naturally lose some of their density and their ability to regrow (remodel) themselves. If you have osteoporosis your bones are much more fragile than they should be, and are much weaker.

Most people don't know they have osteoporosis until it causes them to break a bone. Osteoporosis can make any of your bones more likely to break, but the most commonly affected bones include your:

• Hips (hip fractures).

• Wrists.

• Spine (fractured vertebrae).

The sooner a healthcare provider diagnoses osteoporosis, the less likely you are to experience bone fractures. Ask a healthcare provider about checking your bone density, especially if you're over 65, have had a bone fracture after age 50, or someone in your biological family has osteoporosis.

HOW COMMON IS OSTEOPOROSIS?

More than 50 million people in the U.S. live with osteoporosis. Osteoporosis is common in people over 50. Experts estimate that half of all people assigned female at birth and 1 in 4 people assigned male at birth over 50 have osteoporosis.

Studies have found that 1 in 3 adults over 50 who don't have osteoporosis yet have some degree of reduced bone density (osteopenia). People with osteopenia have early signs of osteoporosis. If it's not treated, osteopenia can become osteoporosis.

Osteoporosis doesn't have symptoms the way lots of other health conditions do. That's why healthcare providers sometimes call it a silent disease. You won't feel or notice anything that signals you might have osteoporosis. You won't have a headache, fever or stomachache that lets you know something in your body is wrong.

The most common "symptom" is suddenly breaking a bone, especially after a small fall or minor accident that usually wouldn't hurt you. Even though osteoporosis doesn't directly cause symptoms, you might notice a few changes in your body that can mean your bones are losing strength or density. These warning signs of osteoporosis can include:

• Losing an inch or more of your height.

• Changes in your natural posture (stooping or bending forward more).

• Shortness of breath (if disks in your spine are compressed enough to reduce your lung capacity).

• Lower back pain (pain in your lumbar spine).

It might be hard to notice changes in your own physical appearance. A loved one may be more likely to see changes in your body (especially your height or posture). People sometimes joke about older adults "shrinking" as they age, but this can be a sign that you should visit a healthcare provider for a bone density test.

WHAT CAUSES OSTEOPOROSIS?

Osteoporosis happens as you get older and your bones lose their ability to regrow and reform themselves. Your bones are living tissue like any other part of your body. It might not seem like it, but they're constantly replacing their own cells and tissue throughout your life. Up until about age 30, your body naturally builds more bone than you lose. After age 35, bone breakdown happens faster than your body can replace it, which causes a gradual loss of bone mass.

If you have osteoporosis, you lose bone mass at a greater rate. People in postmenopause lose bone mass even faster.

Anyone can develop osteoporosis. Some groups of people are more likely to experience it, including:

• Anyone over 50.

• People assigned female at birth (AFAB), especially people AFAB in postmenopause.

• People with a family history (if someone in your biological family has osteoporosis).

• People who are naturally thin or who have "smaller frames." People with thinner statures often have less natural bone mass, so any losses can affect them more.

• People who smoke or use tobacco products.

Some health conditions can make you more likely to develop osteoporosis, including:

• Endocrine disorders — any condition that affects your parathyroid glands, thyroid gland and hormones (like thyroid disease and diabetes).

• Gastrointestinal diseases (like celiac disease and inflammatory bowel disease [IBD]).

• Autoimmune disorders that affect your bones (like rheumatoid arthritis or ankylosing spondylitis — arthritis that affects your spine).

• Blood disorders (or cancers that affect your blood like multiple myeloma).

Some medications or surgical procedures can increase your risk of osteoporosis:

• Diuretics (medications that lower your blood pressure and clear extra fluid from your body.

• Corticosteroids (medications that treat inflammation).

• Medications used to treat seizures.

• Bariatric (weight loss) surgery.

• Hormone therapy for cancer (including to treat breast cancer or prostate cancer).

• Anticoagulants.

• Proton pump inhibitors (like those that treat acid reflux, which can affect your calcium absorption).

Certain aspects of your diet and exercise routine can make you more likely to develop osteoporosis, including:

• Not getting enough calcium or vitamin D in your diet.

• Not getting enough physical exercise.

• Regularly drinking alcohol (more than two drinks per day).

DIAGNOSIS OF OSTEOPOROSIS

The diagnosis of osteoporosis typically involves a combination of medical history assessment, physical examination, and bone density testing. Here's an overview of the diagnostic process:

• Medical History Assessment: Your healthcare provider will begin by asking you about your medical history, including any previous fractures, family history of osteoporosis or fractures, medications you are taking, and lifestyle factors such as smoking and alcohol consumption. They will also inquire about any symptoms you may be experiencing, such as back pain.

• Physical Examination: Your healthcare provider may conduct a physical examination to check for signs of osteoporosis, such as height loss, a curved spine, or poor posture.

• Bone Density Testing: Bone density testing is a key component of the diagnosis of osteoporosis. The most common tests used for this purpose are:

a. Dual-Energy X-ray Absorptiometry (DXA or DEXA): DXA is the gold standard for measuring bone mineral density (BMD). It typically focuses on the hip and spine and provides a T-score, which compares your BMD to that of a young, healthy adult of the same sex. T-scores of -1 and above are considered normal, while scores between -1 and -2.5 indicate low bone mass (osteopenia), and scores of -2.5 or below suggests osteoporosis.

b. Quantitative Ultrasound (QUS): QUS measures bone density at the heel, shin, or finger. While not as widely used as DXA, it can provide an estimate of bone density.

c. Peripheral Dual-Energy X-ray Absorptiometry (pDXA): Similar to DXA, pDXA measures bone density in peripheral sites like the forearm.

• Laboratory Tests: Blood tests may be performed to rule out other medical conditions that could affect bone health. These tests may include measuring calcium levels, vitamin D levels, and markers of bone turnover.

• Fracture Risk Assessment: Your healthcare provider may assess your risk of future fractures using tools like the FRAX (Fracture Risk Assessment Tool) calculator. This tool takes into account factors such as age, sex, bone density, previous fractures, and other risk factors to estimate your ten-year probability of having a major osteoporotic fracture or hip fracture.

• Additional Imaging Studies (Optional): In some cases, additional imaging studies like lateral spine X-rays or vertebral fracture assessment (VFA) may be used to assess the presence of vertebral fractures.

• Special Considerations: In certain situations, additional evaluations may be necessary, such as bone biopsy or genetic testing, particularly if there are atypical features or a suspicion of secondary causes of osteoporosis.

Once a diagnosis of osteoporosis is established, healthcare providers can work with patients to develop a management and treatment plan. This often includes lifestyle modifications, dietary changes, exercise recommendations, and, in some cases, medications to reduce fracture risk and improve bone density. Regular follow-up appointments may also be scheduled to monitor progress and adjust the treatment plan as needed.

TREATMENT OPTIONS

The treatment of osteoporosis aims to reduce the risk of fractures, increase bone density, and manage symptoms associated with the condition. Treatment options for osteoporosis include lifestyle changes, dietary modifications, exercise, and medications. The specific approach chosen depends on the individual's risk factors, bone density measurements, and overall health. Here are the main treatment options for osteoporosis:

1. Lifestyle Modifications:

• Dietary Changes: A diet rich in calcium and vitamin D is essential for bone health. Dairy products, leafy greens, fortified foods, and supplements may be recommended to ensure adequate intake.

• Smoking Cessation: Smoking can contribute to bone loss. Quitting smoking is beneficial for overall health and bone density.

• Limiting Alcohol: Excessive alcohol consumption can weaken bones. Moderation or abstinence is advised.

2. Fall Prevention: Reducing the risk of falls is crucial for individuals with osteoporosis. This may involve removing hazards at home, using assistive devices, and practicing balance exercises.

3. Weight-Bearing Exercise: Engaging in regular weight-bearing and muscle-strengthening exercises helps improve bone density, muscle strength, and balance. Consult with a healthcare provider or physical therapist to develop a safe and effective exercise plan.

4. Medications:

- Bisphosphonates: These drugs, such as alendronate, risedronate, and ibandronate, are commonly prescribed to inhibit bone resorption and increase bone density. They are typically taken orally on a regular schedule.

- Selective Estrogen Receptor Modulators (SERMs): Medications like raloxifene mimic the effects of estrogen on bone density. They are used primarily in postmenopausal women and can reduce the risk of spine fractures.

- Parathyroid Hormone (Teriparatide): Teriparatide is an injectable medication that stimulates bone formation. It is usually prescribed for severe osteoporosis or when other treatments are ineffective.

- Monoclonal Antibody (Denosumab): Denosumab is administered as an injection every six months and works by inhibiting bone resorption. It is an option for individuals who cannot tolerate bisphosphonates or have severe osteoporosis.

- Calcitonin: Calcitonin is available as a nasal spray or injection and can help reduce pain associated with vertebral fractures. It is less commonly used due to its modest effects on bone density.

• Hormone Replacement Therapy (HRT): HRT may be considered for postmenopausal women with severe osteoporosis. It can help maintain bone density but comes with potential risks and benefits that should be discussed with a healthcare provider.

5. Calcium and Vitamin D Supplements: Calcium and vitamin D supplements may be recommended if dietary intake is insufficient. The appropriate dosage varies depending on individual needs and should be determined by a healthcare provider.

6. Fall Prevention Strategies: These include home modifications, such as installing grab bars and removing tripping hazards, wearing appropriate footwear, and using assistive devices like canes or walkers if necessary.

7. Regular Follow-up and Monitoring: Ongoing monitoring is essential to assess treatment effectiveness, check for any potential side effects of medications, and adjust the treatment plan as needed.

The choice of treatment will depend on the severity of osteoporosis, individual risk factors, and patient preferences.

It's crucial to work closely with a healthcare provider to determine the most appropriate treatment strategy for your specific situation. Additionally, lifestyle changes and fall prevention strategies should be incorporated into the management plan to maximize the benefits of treatment and reduce the risk of fractures.

OSTEOPOROSIS AND NUTRITION

Nutrition plays a critical role in managing and preventing osteoporosis, a condition characterized by weakened bones that are more prone to fractures. A balanced diet with the right nutrients can help maintain bone density and overall bone health. Here are some dietary guidelines for osteoporosis:

1. Calcium: Calcium is a crucial mineral for bone health. Aim for the recommended daily intake of calcium, which varies by age and gender but is typically around 1,000-1,300 milligrams per day for adults. Good dietary sources of calcium include dairy products (milk, yogurt, cheese), fortified plant-based milks, leafy greens (kale, collard greens), broccoli, almonds, and canned fish with bones (like salmon and sardines). If it's challenging to get enough calcium from your diet, consider

calcium supplements, but consult with your healthcare provider before starting any supplementation.

2. Vitamin D: Vitamin D is essential for calcium absorption. Spend time in the sun, as your body can produce vitamin D when exposed to sunlight. Aim for 10-30 minutes of sun exposure on your skin several times a week, depending on your location and skin type. Dietary sources of vitamin D include fatty fish (salmon, mackerel), egg yolks, and fortified foods (like fortified milk and breakfast cereals). If you have a vitamin D deficiency, your doctor may recommend supplements.

3. Protein: Adequate protein intake is essential for bone health. Include lean sources of protein like poultry, fish, beans, lentils, tofu, and low-fat dairy products in your diet.

4. Magnesium: Magnesium supports calcium absorption and bone health. Good sources of magnesium include nuts, seeds, whole grains, and leafy greens.

5. Vitamin K: Vitamin K plays a role in bone mineralization. Include dark leafy greens (kale, spinach), broccoli, Brussels sprouts, and other green vegetables in your diet.

6. Phosphorus: Phosphorus is another mineral important for bone health. It's found in dairy products, meat, poultry, fish, and whole grains.

7. Limit Sodium: High sodium intake can lead to calcium loss from bones. Reduce your consumption of processed and salty foods.

8. Limit Caffeine and Alcohol: Excessive caffeine and alcohol consumption can have negative effects on bone health. Limit your intake of caffeinated beverages and alcoholic drinks.

9. Maintain a Healthy Weight: Being underweight can increase the risk of bone loss and fractures. Aim for a healthy body weight through a balanced diet and regular exercise.

10. Omega-3 Fatty Acids: Omega-3 fatty acids, found in fatty fish (like salmon and mackerel) and flaxseeds, may have anti-inflammatory properties that benefit bone health.

11. Fiber: A diet rich in fiber from fruits, vegetables, and whole grains can help with overall health and potentially improve bone density.

It's essential to consult with a healthcare provider or a registered dietitian to create a personalized nutrition plan that takes your specific needs, dietary restrictions, and medical history into account. Additionally, regular bone density testing and check-ups with your healthcare provider are important to monitor your bone health and make necessary adjustments to your diet and lifestyle as needed.

HEALTHY LIFESTYLE CHANGES FOR OSTEOPOROSIS

Making healthy lifestyle changes is crucial for managing and preventing osteoporosis, a condition characterized by weakened bones that are more prone to fractures. Here are some lifestyle changes you can implement to improve bone health and reduce the risk of fractures:

1. Balanced Diet: As mentioned earlier, maintain a diet rich in calcium, vitamin D, protein, magnesium, vitamin K, and phosphorus. Consume plenty of fruits and vegetables for overall health, including bone health. Limit the intake of high-sodium, high-caffeine, and high-alcohol foods and beverages.

2. Regular Exercise: Engage in weight-bearing exercises such as walking, jogging, dancing, and stair climbing to help build and maintain bone density. Incorporate strength training exercises to strengthen muscles and bones. Include balance and flexibility exercises to reduce the risk of falls and fractures. Always warm up before exercising and cool down afterward to prevent injury.

3. Quit Smoking: Smoking can weaken bones and increase the risk of fractures. Seek support and resources to quit smoking if you're a smoker.

4. Limit Alcohol Intake: Excessive alcohol consumption can negatively affect bone health. Aim for moderation or abstain from alcohol, depending on your situation.

5. Fall Prevention: Take measures to prevent falls, as falls can lead to fractures, especially in individuals with osteoporosis. Ensure your home is free from tripping hazards, use handrails on stairs, and install grab bars in the bathroom. Wear supportive footwear with non-slip soles. Have regular vision and hearing check-ups. Consider physical therapy or occupational therapy for balance and fall prevention training.

6. Medication Management: If your healthcare provider prescribes medication to treat or prevent osteoporosis, take it as directed. Discuss the potential side effects and benefits of medications with your healthcare provider.

7. Bone Density Testing: Follow your healthcare provider's recommendations for bone density testing to monitor changes in your bone health.

8. Vitamin and Mineral Supplements: If you have deficiencies in calcium, vitamin D, or other essential nutrients, follow your healthcare provider's guidance on appropriate supplements.

9. Stress Reduction: High levels of stress can have a negative impact on bone health. Engage in stress-reduction techniques such as meditation, yoga, deep breathing exercises, and mindfulness.

10. Regular Check-ups: Schedule regular check-ups with your healthcare provider to monitor your overall health and discuss any concerns related to osteoporosis.

11. Bone-Healthy Lifestyle Education: Stay informed about osteoporosis and bone health through reputable sources and

educational materials. Understanding your condition and its management is essential.

12. Support Groups: Consider joining support groups or seeking the guidance of a healthcare professional who specializes in osteoporosis to connect with others facing similar challenges.

Remember that lifestyle changes may take time to show significant improvements in bone health. It's crucial to work closely with your healthcare provider to develop a personalized plan that considers your specific needs and risk factors. They can provide guidance on the most appropriate lifestyle changes and monitor your progress to ensure you are effectively managing osteoporosis.

OSTEOPOROSIS EXERCISE GUIDE

Exercise is an essential component of managing osteoporosis, a condition characterized by weakened bones that are more susceptible to fractures. The right exercise program can help improve bone density, strengthen muscles, improve balance, and reduce the risk of falls. Here's a guide to exercises for osteoporosis:

Note: Before starting any exercise program, it's crucial to consult with your healthcare provider or a physical therapist, especially if you have severe osteoporosis, other medical conditions, or physical limitations.

• Weight-Bearing Exercises: Weight-bearing exercises put stress on your bones, which helps improve bone density. These exercises can include walking, jogging, hiking, dancing, and stair climbing. Start slowly and gradually increase the intensity and duration of your weight-bearing activities.

• Strength Training: Resistance training helps build muscle strength, which can support and protect your bones. It also improves balance and stability. Use resistance bands, dumbbells, or weight machines for exercises like squats, lunges, leg lifts, bicep curls, and tricep extensions. Perform strength training exercises at least two to three times a week.

• Core and Back Exercises: Strengthening your core and back muscles can improve posture and reduce the risk of vertebral fractures. Exercises like planks, bridges, and seated rows can help strengthen these areas.

• Balance and Posture Exercises: Poor balance and posture can lead to falls and fractures. Incorporate balance exercises into your routine to improve stability. Examples include standing on one leg, heel-to-toe walking, and practicing yoga or tai chi.

• Flexibility and Range of Motion Exercises: Stretching exercises can help maintain flexibility and range of motion, making it easier to perform daily activities. Include gentle stretches for all major muscle groups, focusing on areas prone to tightness.

• Low-Impact Aerobic Exercise: Low-impact activities like swimming and cycling can provide cardiovascular benefits without putting excessive stress on your bones. These exercises are excellent for people who may have joint issues or are unable to engage in high-impact activities.

• Avoid High-Impact Activities: If you have osteoporosis, it's generally best to avoid high-impact activities such as jumping, running on hard surfaces, or participating in contact sports, as they can increase the risk of fractures.

• Breathing Exercises: Breathing exercises can help improve lung function, which is essential for overall health. Practice deep breathing exercises regularly to enhance lung capacity and oxygenation of your body.

• Posture Awareness: Pay attention to your posture during daily activities, such as sitting and standing. Good posture reduces stress on your spine and can help prevent fractures.

• Warm-up and Cool-down: Always start your exercise routine with a proper warm-up and end with a cool-down to prevent injuries.

• Safety Measures:

a. Use proper equipment and footwear during exercise.

b. Ensure your exercise area is clear of tripping hazards.

c. Exercise with a partner or in a supervised environment if necessary.

Remember to progress gradually, and if you experience pain or discomfort during any exercise, stop immediately and consult your healthcare provider. An individualized exercise program designed by a physical therapist or a certified fitness professional with expertise in osteoporosis can be especially beneficial to meet your specific needs and limitations while ensuring safety.

WEIGHT-BEARING EXERCISES

Weight-bearing exercises, also known as weight-bearing or load-bearing activities, are physical activities that involve supporting your body's weight through your bones and muscles. These exercises are excellent for building and maintaining bone density, as they place stress on the bones, stimulating bone growth and strength. Weight-bearing exercises can help reduce the risk of osteoporosis and fractures. Here are some examples of weight-bearing exercises:

• Walking: Walking is a simple yet effective weight-bearing exercise that most people can incorporate into their daily routine. Aim for at least 30 minutes of brisk walking most days of the week.

• Jogging/Running: If you're physically fit and your joints can handle it, jogging or running is a higher-impact form of weight-bearing exercise. Start at a comfortable pace and gradually increase intensity and duration.

• Hiking: Hiking on uneven terrain adds an extra challenge to your bones and muscles. It's a great way to get outdoors and enjoy nature while benefiting your bone health.

• Stair Climbing: Climbing stairs, whether in a building or on a stair-climbing machine, is an effective way to engage your leg muscles and bones.

• Dancing: Dancing, whether it's ballroom, salsa, or even hip-hop, can be an enjoyable weight-bearing exercise that helps improve balance and coordination.

• Aerobic Classes: Joining aerobic classes like step aerobics, Zumba, or dance aerobics can provide a fun way to engage in weight-bearing exercise while also getting a cardio workout.

• Jumping Rope: Jumping rope is a high-impact weight-bearing exercise that can help improve bone density. However, it may not be suitable for everyone, especially those with joint issues.

• Tennis: Racquet sports like tennis, badminton, and pickleball involve quick movements, changes in direction, and impact, making them effective for bone health.

• Team Sports: Many team sports, such as basketball, volleyball, and soccer, involve running, jumping, and quick, dynamic movements that can be beneficial for bones.

• Resistance Training: While not strictly weight-bearing, resistance exercises like weight lifting, bodyweight exercises (e.g., squats, lunges), and resistance band exercises can strengthen the muscles that support your bones, helping to protect against fractures.

When incorporating weight-bearing exercises into your routine, it's important to consider your fitness level, any existing medical conditions, and any joint or mobility issues you may have. If you're new to exercise or have concerns about your bone health, it's a good idea to consult with a healthcare provider or a physical therapist to create a safe and effective exercise plan tailored to your needs and goals. Additionally, remember to start slowly, warm up before exercise, and cool down afterward to prevent injury.

Core and back exercises are essential for maintaining a strong and stable spine, improving posture, reducing the risk of back pain, and enhancing overall physical fitness. Here are some effective core and back exercises you can incorporate into your fitness routine:

Core Exercises:

Plank:

• Start in a push-up position with your arms straight and your hands directly under your shoulders.

• Engage your core muscles and maintain a straight line from head to heels.

• Hold this position for as long as you can, aiming to increase your time gradually.

Side Plank:

• Lie on your side with your legs extended and stack your feet on top of each other.

• Prop yourself up on your elbow, keeping it directly under your shoulder.

• Lift your hips off the ground, forming a straight line from head to heels.

• Hold for as long as you can on each side.

Russian Twists:

• Sit on the floor with your knees bent and your feet flat on the ground.

• Lean back slightly while keeping your back straight and chest up.

• Hold a weight or medicine ball with both hands and twist your torso to the right, bringing the weight beside your right hip.

• Return to the center and then twist to the left. Repeat for the desired number of repetitions.

Leg Raises:

• Lie flat on your back with your arms at your sides and your legs straight.

• Lift your legs off the ground while keeping them straight.

• Lower them back down without touching the ground, then raise them again.

• Continue for the desired number of repetitions.

Bicycle Crunches:

• Lie on your back with your hands behind your head and your knees bent.

• Lift your head, shoulders, and upper back off the ground.

• Bring your right elbow and left knee toward each other while extending your right leg.

• Alternate sides in a pedaling motion.

Back Exercises:

Superman:

• Lie face down with your arms extended in front of you.

• Simultaneously lift your arms, chest, and legs off the ground.

• Hold for a few seconds, then lower back down.

Bridges:

• Lie on your back with your knees bent and feet flat on the floor.

• Lift your hips off the ground, creating a straight line from your shoulders to your knees.

• Squeeze your glutes at the top of the movement, then lower your hips back down.

Deadlifts:

• Use proper form and technique when performing deadlifts with a barbell or dumbbells to strengthen your lower back and hamstrings. Consider seeking guidance from a fitness professional to ensure proper execution.

Lat Pulldowns:

• Use a lat pulldown machine at the gym to target the muscles in your upper back. This exercise can help improve posture and upper body strength.

Seated Rows:

• Perform seated rows using a cable machine or resistance bands to strengthen your middle and upper back.

When performing core and back exercises, focus on maintaining proper form to avoid injury. Start with a weight or resistance level that allows you to complete each exercise with good form, and gradually increase the intensity as you become stronger. It's also a good idea to warm up before these exercises and stretch afterward to prevent muscle tightness and promote flexibility. If you have any existing back conditions or concerns, consult with a healthcare provider or physical therapist before starting a new exercise program.

BALANCE AND POSTURE EXERCISES

Balance and posture exercises are essential for improving stability, preventing falls, reducing the risk of injury, and enhancing overall physical well-being. Incorporating these exercises into your fitness routine can help you maintain better balance and proper posture. Here are some effective balance and posture exercises:

Balance Exercises:

Single-Leg Stance:

• Stand on one leg with the other foot lifted off the ground.

• Try to maintain your balance for as long as possible.

• For an added challenge, close your eyes or stand on an uneven surface like a foam mat.

Heel-to-Toe Walk:

• Walk in a straight line, placing the heel of one foot directly in front of the toes of the other.

• Keep your arms out to the sides for balance.

Balance Board or Wobble Board Exercises:

• Stand on a balance board or wobble board and try to maintain your balance.

• You can also perform exercises like squats or lunges on these boards for added difficulty.

Yoga and Tai Chi:

• Both yoga and tai chi incorporate balance and flexibility exercises into their routines.

• Consider taking a class or following along with online tutorials.

Standing Leg Swings:

• Hold onto a stable surface for support (such as a chair or wall).

• Swing one leg forward and backward while maintaining balance on the other leg.

• Repeat on the other side.

Tandem Stance:

• Stand with one foot in front of the other, heel to toe.

• Hold this position while maintaining balance.

• Switch the position of your feet after a set time.

Posture Exercises:

Wall Angels:

• Stand with your back against a wall and your feet a few inches away from the wall.

• Raise your arms to shoulder height, keeping your elbows and wrists against the wall.

- Slowly slide your arms up and down the wall, trying to maintain contact with the wall throughout the movement.

Chin Tucks:

- Sit or stand with your back straight.

- Gently tuck your chin in toward your chest without tilting your head down.

- Hold for a few seconds and repeat several times.

Cat-Cow Stretch (Yoga):

- Start on your hands and knees in a tabletop position.

- Arch your back (cow) while inhaling and then round your back (cat) while exhaling.

- Repeat this flow several times to improve spinal flexibility and posture.

Thoracic Extension:

- Sit or stand with your back straight.

- Place your hands behind your head and gently arch your upper back to open up the chest.

• Hold for a few seconds and repeat.

Wall Posture Check:

• Stand with your back against a wall, heels about 2-4 inches from the wall.

• Press your lower back, middle back, and the back of your head against the wall.

• Maintain this position while performing daily tasks to reinforce good posture.

Incorporate these balance and posture exercises into your fitness routine a few times a week. Gradually increase the intensity and duration as your balance and posture improve. Remember to practice these exercises with proper form and alignment to maximize their benefits and reduce the risk of injury. If you have specific posture concerns or any existing musculoskeletal issues, consider consulting a physical therapist or fitness professional for guidance tailored to your needs.

FLEXIBILITY AND RANGE OF MOTION EXERCISES

Flexibility and range of motion (ROM) exercises are essential for maintaining joint health, preventing stiffness, and improving overall mobility. Incorporating these exercises into your daily routine can help increase your flexibility and allow you to move more comfortably. Here are some effective flexibility and ROM exercises:

Neck Stretches:

• Gently tilt your head to the right, bringing your ear toward your shoulder.

• Hold for 15-30 seconds, then switch sides.

• Perform forward and backward neck stretches by tilting your head forward and backward.

Shoulder Rolls:

• Roll your shoulders forward in a circular motion for 10-15 seconds.

• Reverse the motion by rolling your shoulders backward for another 10-15 seconds.

Arm Circles:

• Stand with your feet shoulder-width apart and extend your arms straight out to the sides.

• Make small circles with your arms, gradually increasing the size of the circles.

• After 20-30 seconds, reverse the direction of the circles.

Trunk Twists:

• Sit or stand with your feet hip-width apart.

• Twist your upper body to the right while keeping your hips facing forward.

• Hold for 15-30 seconds, then twist to the left.

Cat-Cow Stretch (Yoga):

• Start on your hands and knees in a tabletop position.

• Arch your back (cow) while inhaling and then round your back (cat) while exhaling.

• Repeat this flow several times to improve spinal flexibility.

Seated Forward Bend:

• Sit with your legs extended straight in front of you.

• Reach forward toward your toes while keeping your back straight.

• Hold for 15-30 seconds while breathing deeply.

Hip Flexor Stretch:

• Kneel on one knee with your other foot in front, forming a 90-degree angle with your knee.

• Push your hips forward slightly until you feel a stretch in the front of your hip.

• Hold for 15-30 seconds, then switch sides.

Quadriceps Stretch:

• Stand on one leg and bend your other knee, bringing your heel toward your buttocks.

• Hold your ankle with your hand to deepen the stretch.

• Hold for 15-30 seconds, then switch legs.

Calf Stretch:

• Stand facing a wall with one foot forward and one foot back.

• Lean forward, keeping your back leg straight and your heel on the ground.

• Hold for 15-30 seconds, then switch legs.

Ankle Circles:

• Sit on a chair or the floor with your legs extended.

• Rotate your ankles in a circular motion for 20-30 seconds in each direction.

Wrist Flexor and Extensor Stretches:

• Extend one arm straight in front of you.

• With your other hand, gently bend your wrist forward (flexor stretch) and backward (extensor stretch) for 15-30 seconds each.

Perform these flexibility and ROM exercises regularly to maintain and improve your joint mobility. Always start with a gentle warm-up to prepare your muscles and joints for stretching, and perform each stretch slowly and smoothly without bouncing. If you have specific mobility concerns or limitations, consult a physical therapist or fitness professional for guidance tailored to your needs.

LOW-IMPACT AEROBIC EXERCISE

Low-impact aerobic exercises are excellent choices for individuals who want to improve cardiovascular fitness, burn calories, and maintain overall health without putting excessive stress on the joints. These exercises are particularly suitable for those with joint issues, arthritis, or other conditions that limit high-impact activities. Here are some low-impact aerobic exercises you can consider incorporating into your fitness routine:

• Walking: Walking is one of the most accessible and effective low-impact exercises. It can be done indoors on a treadmill or outdoors in your neighborhood or at a local park. To increase intensity, you can add hills or increase your pace.

• Swimming: Swimming and water aerobics are excellent choices for low-impact cardio workouts. The buoyancy of the water reduces stress on the joints while providing a full-body workout.

• Cycling: Riding a stationary bike or a regular bicycle on flat terrain is a low-impact way to improve cardiovascular fitness. Many fitness centers offer stationary cycling classes.

• Elliptical Trainer: Elliptical machines provide a low-impact workout that mimics the motion of walking or running without the impact on the joints. These machines often have handlebars for a full-body workout.

• Rowing: Using a rowing machine engages multiple muscle groups and provides a low-impact cardio workout. It's especially effective for working the upper body.

• Dancing: Low-impact dance styles like ballroom, salsa, and tango can be a fun way to get your heart rate up without stressing your joints. Consider taking dance classes or following online tutorials.

• Aerobic Step Classes: Low-impact step aerobics classes use a step platform to provide a cardio workout without high-impact movements. The step height can be adjusted to match your fitness level.

• Group Fitness Classes: Many fitness centers offer group classes like low-impact aerobics, Pilates, and yoga, which can provide cardiovascular benefits without the impact on your joints.

• Tai Chi: This gentle martial art combines slow, flowing movements with deep breathing and meditation. It improves balance, flexibility, and cardiovascular fitness in a low-impact manner.

• Mini Trampoline (Rebounding): Bouncing on a mini trampoline can provide a low-impact aerobic workout that is easy on the joints. Make sure to use proper form and start with gentle bounces.

• Seated Exercises: If you have difficulty standing or balancing, seated exercises can provide a low-impact cardio workout. Consider exercises like seated leg lifts, seated marches, or seated dancing.

When engaging in low-impact aerobic exercises, remember to start slowly and gradually increase the duration and intensity of your workouts. Pay attention to proper form and technique to avoid injury. Additionally, consult with a healthcare provider or fitness professional, especially if you have any underlying medical conditions or physical limitations, to ensure that your exercise program is safe and appropriate for your needs.

STRENGTH TRAINING FOR OSTEOPOROSIS

Strength training, also known as resistance training or weight lifting, is highly beneficial for individuals with osteoporosis. It helps build and maintain muscle mass, improve bone density, and reduce the risk of fractures by strengthening the bones and surrounding muscles. Here's a guide to strength training for osteoporosis:

• Consult Your Healthcare Provider: Before starting any strength training program, consult with your healthcare provider to ensure that it is safe and appropriate for your individual condition.

• Seek Guidance: Consider working with a certified fitness professional or physical therapist who has experience with osteoporosis. They can design a personalized exercise plan and provide proper guidance.

• Start with a Warm-up: Begin your strength training routine with a 5-10 minutes warm-up to increase blood flow to your muscles and prepare your body for exercise. Activities like light cardio or dynamic stretching can be effective.

• Choose the Right Equipment: You can use free weights, resistance bands, weight machines, or your body weight for strength training. Resistance bands are often recommended for their versatility and adaptability to various fitness levels.

• Focus on Proper Form: Maintaining proper form is crucial to prevent injuries and get the most benefit from your exercises. Start with light weights or resistance and ensure you can perform each exercise with good form before increasing the resistance.

• Target Major Muscle Groups: A well-rounded strength training program should include exercises that target the major muscle groups of the body. These typically include:

a. Chest: Bench press, push-ups

b. Back: Rows, lat pulldowns

c. Legs: Squats, lunges, leg presses

d. Hips and Glutes: Hip bridges, leg lifts

e. Shoulders: Dumbbell or resistance band shoulder presses

f. Core: Planks, stability ball exercises

• Progressive Overload: To see improvements in bone density and muscle strength, gradually increase the resistance or weight as your muscles adapt to the exercises.

• Sets and Repetitions: Aim for 2-3 sets of 8-12 repetitions per exercise. Allow for 48 hours of rest between sessions targeting the same muscle group.

• Breathing: Exhale during the lifting phase of the exercise and inhale during the lowering phase.

• Safety Precautions: Avoid exercises that involve bending at the waist, twisting the spine, or high-impact activities. Maintain proper spine alignment during all exercises. Use a stable chair or bench for seated exercises. If you experience pain or discomfort while performing an exercise, stop immediately and consult with your healthcare provider or fitness professional.

• Cool Down: Finish your strength training session with a cool-down period, which can include stretching exercises to improve flexibility and reduce muscle soreness.

• Consistency is Key: Aim to strength train at least 2-3 times per week to see improvements in bone density and muscle strength over time.

Strength training for osteoporosis can significantly enhance bone health and overall physical well-being when done correctly and safely. Remember that it's essential to work with a healthcare provider or fitness professional to tailor your strength training program to your specific needs and to monitor your progress over time.

BREATHING EXERCISES

Breathing exercises can be a valuable tool for managing stress, improving lung function, enhancing relaxation, and even boosting overall well-being. Here are several breathing exercises that you can practice to achieve various benefits:

Deep Abdominal Breathing (Diaphragmatic Breathing):

• Sit or lie down in a comfortable position.

• Place one hand on your chest and the other on your abdomen.

• Inhale deeply through your nose, allowing your abdomen to rise (your chest should remain relatively still).

• Exhale slowly and completely through your mouth or nose.

• Focus on making your breaths slow, deep, and controlled.

4-7-8 Breathing (Relaxing Breath):

• Sit or lie down in a comfortable position.

• Close your eyes and take a deep breath in through your nose for a count of 4.

• Hold your breath for a count of 7.

• Exhale slowly and completely through your mouth for a count of 8.

• Repeat this cycle several times.

Box Breathing (Four-Square Breathing):

• Sit in a relaxed position.

• Inhale for a count of 4.

• Hold your breath for a count of 4.

• Exhale for a count of 4.

• Hold your breath for a count of 4.

• Repeat this cycle as needed.

Alternate Nostril Breathing (Nadi Shodhana):

• Sit comfortably with your back straight.

• Use your right thumb to close your right nostril and your right ring finger to close your left nostril.

• Close your eyes and take a deep breath in through your left nostril.

• Close your left nostril with your ring finger and release your right nostril.

• Exhale through your right nostril.

• Inhale through your right nostril.

• Close your right nostril with your thumb and release your left nostril.

• Exhale through your left nostril.

• Repeat this cycle, alternating nostrils for several rounds.

Breath Counting:

• Sit quietly and comfortably.

• Inhale and exhale naturally.

• Count each complete breath cycle (one inhale and one exhale) up to a specified number (e.g., 10).

• If your mind wanders or you lose count, gently return to counting without judgment.

3-Part Breath (Yogic Full Breath):

• Sit or lie down comfortably.

• Begin by inhaling deeply into your abdomen, feeling it expand.

• Continue the inhalation into your ribcage, expanding your chest.

• Finally, breathe into your upper chest and throat.

• Exhale slowly and completely in reverse order (first from the throat, then chest, and finally the abdomen).

• Visualize your breath moving through these three parts of your body.

Guided Visualization with Breath:

• Close your eyes and take several deep breaths to relax.

• Visualize a peaceful place or a situation that brings you joy and contentment.

• Sync your breathing with this visualization, inhaling positive energy and exhaling any stress or tension.

Breathing exercises can be performed anytime, anywhere, and they are especially effective when practiced regularly. You can use these techniques to manage stress, promote relaxation, improve focus, or enhance mindfulness. Experiment with different exercises to find the ones that resonate with you the most and incorporate them into your daily routine as needed. If you have specific health concerns or breathing difficulties, consult with a healthcare provider or a qualified breathing coach for guidance and personalized recommendations.

EFFECT OF HIGH IMPACT ACTIVITIES ON OSTEOPOROSIS PATIENTS

High-impact activities can have both positive and negative effects on individuals with osteoporosis, depending on several factors, including the person's bone health, overall fitness level, and the safety precautions taken. It's important for individuals with osteoporosis to carefully consider the impact of high-impact activities and, in many cases, consult with a healthcare provider before engaging in them. Here are some key points to consider:

Positive Effects of High-Impact Activities:

• Bone Density Improvement: High-impact activities can stimulate bone growth and increase bone density. These activities put stress on the bones, which can trigger the body's natural bone-building process.

• Muscle Strength and Balance: Many high-impact activities also involve strength and balance components. Strengthening muscles and improving balance can reduce the risk of falls and fractures.

• Cardiovascular Benefits: High-impact activities often provide an excellent cardiovascular workout, which is essential for overall health. Improved cardiovascular fitness can reduce the risk of heart disease and improve general well-being.

Negative Effects of High-Impact Activities:

• Risk of Fractures: Individuals with severe osteoporosis or those who have already experienced fractures may be at risk for further fractures when engaging in high-impact activities. Fragile bones may not withstand the impact, leading to injuries.

• Joint Stress: High-impact activities can stress the joints, particularly the knees, hips, and spine. This can be problematic for individuals with joint issues or arthritis in addition to osteoporosis.

• Safety Concerns: Safety is a significant concern when participating in high-impact activities. Falls and improper technique can lead to injuries, especially for those with compromised bone health.

Considerations for High-Impact Activities:

If you have osteoporosis and are considering high-impact activities, it's essential to follow these guidelines:

• Consult with Your Healthcare Provider: Before starting any high-impact exercise program, discuss your plans with your healthcare provider. They can assess your bone health and provide personalized recommendations.

• Bone Density Testing: Regular bone density testing can help monitor your progress and identify any changes in your bone health.

• Gradual Progression: If your healthcare provider approves, start slowly and gradually increase the intensity and duration of your high-impact activities.

• Proper Technique: Ensure that you learn proper technique for high-impact exercises to minimize the risk of injury.

• Consider Low-Impact Alternatives: In some cases, low-impact or moderate-impact activities may be a safer option.

Activities like walking, swimming, and cycling provide cardiovascular benefits without as much impact on the joints.

• Use Protective Gear: If appropriate, consider using protective gear, such as knee or wrist braces, to reduce the risk of injury.

• Listen to Your Body: Pay close attention to how your body responds to high-impact activities. If you experience pain, discomfort, or other concerning symptoms, stop the activity and seek medical advice.

Ultimately, whether high-impact activities are suitable for individuals with osteoporosis depends on individual factors and the stage of the disease. Safety should always be a top priority, and any exercise program should be tailored to the individual's specific needs and capabilities. Consulting with a healthcare provider and, if necessary, a qualified fitness professional can help you make informed decisions about your exercise routine.

IMPORTANCE OF EXERCISES FOR OSTEOPOROSIS

Exercise plays a crucial role in the management and prevention of osteoporosis. Here are several key reasons why exercise is important for individuals with osteoporosis:

• Improves Bone Density: Weight-bearing exercises and resistance training stimulate the bones to become denser and stronger. This helps counteract the bone loss associated with osteoporosis, making the bones less prone to fractures.

• Strengthens Muscles: Exercise helps build and maintain muscle mass. Strong muscles provide support to the bones, reducing the risk of falls and fractures.

• Enhances Balance and Coordination: Many exercise programs, including balance and posture exercises like yoga and tai chi, improve stability and coordination. This is particularly important for individuals with osteoporosis, as it reduces the likelihood of falls.

• Reduces the Risk of Falls: Regular exercise can improve overall physical fitness and agility, making it easier to react quickly and maintain balance when faced with a potentially hazardous situation. This reduces the risk of falls, which can lead to fractures in individuals with fragile bones.

• Increases Joint Mobility: Exercises that focus on flexibility and range of motion help maintain joint health. This can enhance overall mobility and reduce the risk of injuries caused by stiff or restricted joints.

• Promotes Good Posture: Exercises that strengthen the core and back muscles can improve posture and reduce the risk of vertebral fractures, a common complication of osteoporosis.

• Boosts Cardiovascular Health: Cardiovascular exercises, such as walking and swimming, improve heart and lung health. Cardiovascular fitness is essential for overall well-being and can enhance your ability to engage in daily activities.

• Enhances Mental Well-being: Exercise has been shown to reduce stress, anxiety, and depression. These mental health benefits can be particularly important for individuals with osteoporosis, as the condition can be emotionally challenging.

• Supports Weight Management: Regular exercise can help with weight management or weight loss, which is important because excessive body weight can place additional stress on the bones and increase the risk of fractures.

• Improves Quality of Life: Engaging in physical activity can enhance one's overall quality of life. It promotes independence, allows for greater participation in daily activities, and helps individuals maintain an active and fulfilling lifestyle.

It's essential to note that the type and intensity of exercise should be tailored to an individual's specific condition, age, and fitness level. Consulting with a healthcare provider or physical therapist is crucial to ensure that the chosen exercise program is safe and appropriate. Additionally, gradual progression of exercise and proper technique are important to prevent injuries. By incorporating regular, appropriately tailored exercise into their routines, individuals with osteoporosis can significantly improve their bone health and overall well-being.

ADVANTAGES OF LOW IMPACT ACTIVITIES FOR OSTEOPOROSIS

Low-impact activities offer several advantages for individuals with osteoporosis. These activities are gentler on the joints and bones while providing numerous health benefits. Here are the advantages of low-impact activities for osteoporosis:

• Reduced Risk of Fractures: Low-impact activities are less likely to cause fractures or injuries in individuals with fragile bones. High-impact exercises can put excessive stress on bones and increase the risk of fractures, especially if the individual already has osteoporosis.

• Improved Bone Health: While low-impact activities may not stimulate bone growth as effectively as high-impact exercises, they still provide some benefit by maintaining bone density. Consistent low-impact exercise can help slow down the rate of bone loss.

• Joint Protection: Low-impact activities are easier on the joints, making them suitable for individuals with joint issues or arthritis, which can often coexist with osteoporosis. These activities can help maintain joint health and reduce the risk of joint pain.

• Enhanced Cardiovascular Fitness: Low-impact aerobic exercises like swimming, water aerobics, and stationary cycling offer cardiovascular benefits without the impact stress on the joints. They can help improve heart and lung health.

• Improved Balance and Coordination: Low-impact activities that incorporate balance and stability, such as yoga and tai chi, can help improve balance and reduce the risk of falls and fractures. Better balance is especially important for those with osteoporosis.

• Gradual Progression: Low-impact exercises are typically easier to start for beginners or individuals who have been sedentary. They allow for gradual progression and adaptation as fitness levels improve.

• Long-Term Sustainability: Low-impact activities can often be maintained over the long term, making them suitable for individuals looking to establish a sustainable exercise routine that they can continue as they age.

• Pain Management: For individuals with chronic pain or discomfort associated with osteoporosis, low-impact activities can be more comfortable and less likely to exacerbate existing pain.

• Reduced Stress: Engaging in low-impact exercises can have a calming effect on the body and mind, reducing stress and promoting relaxation, which is important for overall well-being.

• Versatility: Low-impact activities encompass a wide range of options, including walking, swimming, stationary cycling, elliptical training, and low-impact aerobics. This variety allows individuals to choose activities that align with their preferences and limitations.

It's important to note that while low-impact activities offer these advantages, they may not provide the same level of bone-strengthening benefits as high-impact exercises. Therefore, a well-rounded exercise routine may include a combination of both low-impact and weight-bearing activities to maximize bone health while minimizing the risk of injury. Before starting any exercise program, individuals with osteoporosis should consult with a healthcare provider or physical therapist to ensure that their chosen activities are safe and appropriate for their specific condition.

PART TWO

BREAKFAST RECIPES

Cottage Cheese Pancakes

Ingredients:

• 1 cup cottage cheese (low-fat or full-fat, as per your preference)

• 4 large eggs

• 1/4 cup all-purpose flour (or whole wheat flour for a healthier option)

• 1/4 teaspoon baking powder

• 1 tablespoon sugar or honey (optional, for sweetness)

• 1/2 teaspoon vanilla extract (optional)

• Pinch of salt

• Cooking oil or butter for the skillet

Instructions:

1. In a blender or food processor, combine the cottage cheese, eggs, flour, baking powder, sugar or honey (if using), vanilla extract (if using), and a pinch of salt. Blend or process until you have a smooth batter. Alternatively, you can mix these ingredients in a bowl using a hand mixer or whisk.

2. Preheat a non-stick skillet or griddle over medium heat. Add a small amount of cooking oil or butter and spread it evenly to prevent sticking.

3. Pour small portions of the pancake batter onto the skillet to form pancakes of your desired size. You can make them small for mini pancakes or larger for traditional-sized pancakes.

4. Cook the pancakes until you see bubbles forming on the surface, which usually takes about 2-3 minutes.

5. Carefully flip the pancakes using a spatula and cook the other side for another 2-3 minutes, or until they are golden brown and cooked through.

6. Continue making pancakes with the remaining batter, adding more oil or butter to the skillet as needed.

7. Serve the cottage cheese pancakes hot. You can garnish them with fresh fruit, a dollop of Greek yogurt, a drizzle of honey or maple syrup, or a sprinkle of powdered sugar, as desired.

8. Enjoy your protein-rich and flavorful cottage cheese pancakes for a satisfying breakfast.

Veggie Breakfast Burrito

Ingredients:

For the Burrito Filling:

• 1/2 cup diced bell peppers (any color)

• 1/2 cup diced onions

• 1/2 cup diced tomatoes

• 1/2 cup sliced mushrooms

• 1/2 cup spinach or kale, chopped

• 1/2 cup cooked black beans (canned or cooked from dry)

• 4 large eggs (or use tofu for a vegan option)

• Salt and pepper to taste

• Olive oil for sautéing

For Assembling:

• 4 large whole wheat or spinach tortillas

• Salsa or hot sauce (optional)

• Shredded cheese (optional, use vegan cheese if preferred)

• Fresh cilantro or parsley for garnish (optional)

Instructions:

1. Dice the bell peppers, onions, tomatoes, and mushrooms. Chop the spinach or kale. Rinse and drain the black beans if using canned.

2. In a large skillet, heat a tablespoon of olive oil over medium heat. Add the diced onions and cook until they become translucent, about 2-3 minutes.

3. Add the diced bell peppers and sliced mushrooms. Sauté until they start to soften, about 3-4 minutes. Stir in the diced tomatoes and cook for an additional 2 minutes. Add the

chopped spinach or kale and cook until wilted, about 1-2 minutes.

4. Finally, add the cooked black beans to the skillet and heat them through. Season the vegetable mixture with salt and pepper to taste. Set aside.

5. In a separate bowl, whisk the eggs (or crumble tofu for a vegan option). Season with salt and pepper. In the same skillet you used for the vegetables, add a bit more oil if needed. Pour in the whisked eggs (or crumbled tofu) and scramble them until cooked to your liking. Remove from heat.

6. Lay out the tortillas on a clean surface. Divide the cooked vegetable mixture and scrambled eggs (or tofu) evenly among the tortillas.

7. If desired, sprinkle shredded cheese over the filling for added flavor. Fold in the sides of each tortilla, then roll it up tightly from the bottom to create a burrito shape.

8. Place the veggie breakfast burritos seam-side down on a plate. You can serve them as they are or cut them in half diagonally for easier eating.

9. If you like, garnish your burritos with fresh cilantro or parsley, and serve with salsa or hot sauce on the side.

Salmon and Cream Cheese Bagel

Ingredients:

• 1 bagel (your choice of flavor)

• 2-3 tablespoons cream cheese (plain or flavored, like chive or herb)

• 2-3 slices of smoked salmon

• Thinly sliced red onion (optional)

• Capers (optional)

• Fresh dill sprigs (optional)

• Lemon wedges (optional)

• Salt and black pepper to taste

Instructions:

1. Slice the bagel in half horizontally. Toast it until it reaches your desired level of crispiness. You can use a toaster or oven for this step.

2. Once the bagel is toasted, spread a generous layer of cream cheese on both halves. You can use plain cream cheese or choose a flavored variety for added flavor.

3. Lay the slices of smoked salmon evenly on the bottom half of the bagel. The cream cheese will act as a creamy base for the salmon.

4. If you like, you can add thinly sliced red onion rings, capers, and a sprig or two of fresh dill for extra flavor and garnish.

5. Sprinkle a pinch of salt and a dash of black pepper over the salmon for seasoning. Place the top half of the bagel over the salmon to create a sandwich.

6. Your salmon and cream cheese bagel is ready to serve. You can serve it as a whole sandwich or cut it in half diagonally for a more elegant presentation.

7. If desired, garnish your bagel with additional fresh dill sprigs and serve with lemon wedges on the side. Squeezing a bit of lemon juice over the salmon can enhance the flavors.

8. Enjoy your delicious salmon and cream cheese bagel for breakfast, brunch, or as a satisfying snack.

Pumpkin and Chia Seed Porridge

Ingredients:

• Rolled oats

• Canned pumpkin puree

• Chia seeds

• Pumpkin pie spice

• Sliced bananas

Instructions:

1. Cook rolled oats with canned pumpkin puree, chia seeds, and a sprinkle of pumpkin pie spice.

2. Top with sliced bananas.

Salmon and Spinach Breakfast Wrap

Ingredients:

• Whole-grain tortilla

• Smoked salmon

• Sautéed spinach

• Scrambled eggs

• Low-fat cream cheese

Instructions:

1. Spread low-fat cream cheese on a whole-grain tortilla.

2. Layer with smoked salmon, sautéed spinach, and scrambled eggs.

3. Roll up the tortilla into a wrap.

Peach and Walnut Yogurt Parfait

Ingredients:

• Low-fat yogurt

- Sliced peaches (canned or fresh)

- Chopped walnuts

- Ground cinnamon

Instructions:

1. In a glass, layer low-fat yogurt, sliced peaches, and chopped walnuts.

2. Sprinkle with a pinch of ground cinnamon.

Chia Seed Pudding with Almonds and Berries

Ingredients:

- Chia seeds

- Almond milk

- Sliced almonds

- Mixed berries

- Honey (optional)

Instructions:

1. Mix chia seeds and almond milk in a jar, and refrigerate overnight.

2. In the morning, top with sliced almonds, mixed berries, and a drizzle of honey.

Broccoli and Cheese Frittata

Ingredients:

• Eggs

• Chopped broccoli florets

• Shredded low-fat cheese

• Chopped onions

• Olive oil

Instructions:

• Sauté chopped broccoli and onions in olive oil until tender.

• Pour beaten eggs over the veggies, sprinkle with shredded cheese, and cook until set.

Berry and Spinach Smoothie Bowl

Ingredients:

• Frozen mixed berries

• Fresh spinach leaves

• Greek yogurt

• Almond milk

• Ground flaxseed

Instructions:

1. Blend frozen berries, spinach, Greek yogurt, almond milk, and ground flaxseed until smooth.

2. Pour into a bowl and top with additional berries or granola if desired.

Oat Bran Pancakes

Ingredients:

• Oat bran

• Whole-wheat flour

- Baking powder

- Low-fat milk

- Egg whites

Instructions:

1. Mix oat bran, whole-wheat flour, and baking powder in a bowl.

2. Add low-fat milk and egg whites to create a pancake batter.

3. Cook pancakes on a griddle until golden brown.

Tomato and Basil Breakfast Sandwich

Ingredients:

- Whole-grain English muffin

- Sliced tomatoes

- Fresh basil leaves

- Poached or fried egg

- Low-fat mozzarella cheese

Instructions:

1. Toast a whole-grain English muffin.

2. Layer with sliced tomatoes, fresh basil leaves, a poached or fried egg, and low-fat mozzarella cheese.

Greek Yogurt Parfait with Nuts and Berries

Ingredients:

• Greek yogurt

• Mixed berries (e.g., strawberries, blueberries, raspberries)

• Chopped nuts (e.g., almonds, walnuts)

• Honey (optional)

Instructions:

1. In a glass or bowl, layer Greek yogurt, mixed berries, and chopped nuts.

2. Drizzle with honey if desired.

3. Enjoy this calcium and protein-rich parfait.

Spinach and Feta Omelette

Ingredients:

- Eggs

- Chopped spinach

- Crumbled feta cheese

- Chopped tomatoes

- Chopped onions

- Olive oil

Instructions:

1. In a bowl, beat eggs with a pinch of salt and pepper.

2. In a non-stick skillet, sauté chopped spinach, chopped tomatoes, and chopped onions in olive oil until softened.

3. Pour beaten eggs over the vegetables and cook until set.

4. Sprinkle crumbled feta cheese on one half of the omelette, fold it over, and serve.

Oatmeal with Almond Butter and Banana

Ingredients:

• Rolled oats

• Almond butter

• Sliced bananas

• Chopped almonds

• Cinnamon

• Honey (optional)

Instructions:

1. Cook rolled oats with water or milk according to package instructions.

2. Top the oatmeal with almond butter, sliced bananas, chopped almonds, and a sprinkle of cinnamon.

3. Drizzle with honey if desired.

Whole-Grain Pancakes with Blueberries

Ingredients:

- Whole-grain pancake mix

- Fresh or frozen blueberries

- Low-fat yogurt

- Maple syrup (optional)

Instructions:

1. Prepare whole-grain pancake batter according to the package instructions.

2. Add fresh or frozen blueberries to the batter.

3. Cook pancakes on a griddle or skillet until golden brown.

4. Serve with a dollop of low-fat yogurt and a drizzle of maple syrup if desired.

Tofu Scramble

Ingredients:

- 1 block of firm tofu (about 14 oz)

- 1-2 tablespoons olive oil or cooking oil of your choice

- 1/2 cup diced onions

- 1/2 cup diced bell peppers (any color)

- 1/2 cup diced tomatoes

- 1/2 cup sliced mushrooms

- 1/2 cup spinach or kale, chopped

- 1-2 cloves garlic, minced

- 1/2 teaspoon turmeric powder (for color)

- 1/2 teaspoon cumin powder

- 1/2 teaspoon paprika (smoked or sweet)

- Salt and pepper to taste

- Optional toppings: avocado, diced avocado, hot sauce, nutritional yeast, chopped fresh herbs

Instructions:

1. Remove the tofu from its packaging and drain any excess liquid. Place the tofu block on a clean kitchen towel or paper towels. Press gently to remove more moisture.

2. Crumble the tofu into small, bite-sized pieces using your hands or a fork. Aim for a scrambled egg-like consistency. Set aside.

3. In a large skillet, heat the olive oil over medium heat. Add the diced onions and sauté for 2-3 minutes until they become translucent.

4. Stir in the minced garlic, turmeric powder (for color), cumin powder, and paprika. Sauté for an additional 30 seconds until the spices become fragrant.

5. Add the diced bell peppers, sliced mushrooms, and chopped tomatoes to the skillet. Sauté for 3-4 minutes until the vegetables start to soften.

6. Add the crumbled tofu to the skillet, and gently fold it into the sautéed vegetables. Cook for another 3-4 minutes, allowing the tofu to heat through.

7. Add the chopped spinach or kale to the skillet. Cook for a few more minutes until the greens wilt and the tofu is heated thoroughly. Stir occasionally.

8. Season the tofu scramble with salt and pepper to taste. Taste and adjust the seasonings or spices as needed to suit your preferences.

9. Serve your tofu scramble hot. You can top it with diced avocado, a drizzle of hot sauce, a sprinkle of nutritional yeast for a cheesy flavor (if desired), or chopped fresh herbs like parsley or cilantro.

10. Serve your tofu scramble as a delicious and satisfying breakfast or brunch option.

Overnight Chia Pudding

Ingredients:

• 1/4 cup chia seeds

• 1 cup milk (dairy or non-dairy like almond milk, coconut milk, or soy milk)

• 1-2 tablespoons sweetener of your choice (e.g., honey, maple syrup, agave nectar)

• 1/2 teaspoon vanilla extract (optional)

• Fresh fruits (e.g., berries, sliced banana) for topping

- Nuts (e.g., almonds, walnuts) for topping (optional)

- Unsweetened shredded coconut or cocoa nibs for topping (optional)

Instructions:

1. In a mixing bowl or a jar with a lid, combine the chia seeds and your choice of milk. Stir well to evenly distribute the chia seeds in the liquid.

2. Stir in the sweetener of your choice (e.g., honey, maple syrup) and vanilla extract if you'd like to add extra flavor.

3. Stir the mixture again after a few minutes to prevent clumping, then cover it and refrigerate. It's essential to refrigerate the chia pudding for at least a few hours or, ideally, overnight to allow the chia seeds to absorb the liquid and create a pudding-like consistency.

4. You can check the pudding after an hour or so and give it a good stir to ensure the chia seeds are evenly distributed. This step is optional but can help prevent clumping.

5. Once the chia pudding has thickened to your desired consistency, usually after several hours or overnight, it's ready to serve.

6. Spoon the chia pudding into serving bowls or jars. Top it with fresh fruits like berries or sliced banana, nuts for added crunch, and optional toppings like shredded coconut or cocoa nibs.

7. Feel free to customize your chia pudding with your favorite toppings, spices (e.g., cinnamon), or additional flavorings (e.g., almond extract). You can also layer it with yogurt or granola for added texture.

Quinoa Breakfast Bowl

Ingredients:

For the Quinoa:

• 1 cup quinoa

• 2 cups water

• Pinch of salt

For Assembling:

• Greek yogurt (plain or flavored)

• Fresh mixed berries (e.g., strawberries, blueberries, raspberries)

• Sliced banana

• Nuts and seeds (e.g., almonds, walnuts, chia seeds)

• Honey or maple syrup for drizzling (optional)

• Cinnamon or nutmeg for sprinkling (optional)

Instructions:

1. Rinse the quinoa thoroughly under cold running water to remove any bitterness. In a medium saucepan, combine the rinsed quinoa, water, and a pinch of salt. Bring it to a boil.

2. Reduce the heat to low, cover the saucepan, and let the quinoa simmer for about 15-20 minutes, or until all the water is absorbed and the quinoa is tender. Remove it from heat.

3. Fluff the cooked quinoa with a fork to separate the grains. Let it cool slightly before assembling your breakfast bowl. You can

also make the quinoa ahead of time and store it in the refrigerator.

4. In a serving bowl, start with a portion of cooked quinoa as the base.

5. Add a generous dollop of Greek yogurt on top of the quinoa. Greek yogurt adds creaminess and extra protein to your bowl.

6. Layer fresh mixed berries and sliced banana over the yogurt. You can use any combination of berries you like.

7. Sprinkle a handful of nuts and seeds over the top for added crunch, healthy fats, and nutrients. Chopped almonds, walnuts, and chia seeds are great choices.

8. If you prefer a touch of sweetness, drizzle honey or maple syrup over the ingredients. You can adjust the amount to your taste.

9. For extra flavor, sprinkle a pinch of cinnamon or nutmeg over the top. Your quinoa breakfast bowl is ready to serve. Enjoy it as a nutritious and satisfying breakfast or brunch option.

Peanut Butter Banana Smoothie

Ingredients:

• 1 ripe banana

• 2 tablespoons peanut butter (creamy or crunchy, as you prefer)

• 1 cup milk (dairy or non-dairy like almond milk, soy milk, or oat milk)

• 1/2 cup plain Greek yogurt (optional, for added creaminess and protein)

• 1-2 tablespoons honey or maple syrup (optional, for added sweetness)

• 1/2 teaspoon vanilla extract (optional)

• A pinch of salt (optional)

• Ice cubes (optional, for a colder smoothie)

Instructions:

1. Peel the ripe banana and break it into smaller chunks. This makes it easier to blend.

2. Place the banana chunks, peanut butter, milk, Greek yogurt (if using), honey or maple syrup (if using), vanilla extract (if using), and a pinch of salt (if using) into a blender.

3. If you prefer a colder and thicker smoothie, you can add a handful of ice cubes to the blender.

4. Blend all the ingredients until you have a smooth and creamy consistency. This usually takes about 1-2 minutes.

5. Taste the smoothie and adjust the sweetness or thickness as needed. You can add more honey, peanut butter, or milk to suit your preferences. Pour the peanut butter banana smoothie into a glass or to-go cup.

6. For an extra touch, you can garnish your smoothie with a drizzle of peanut butter, banana slices, or a sprinkle of crushed peanuts.

7. Your delicious peanut butter banana smoothie is ready to enjoy. Sip it as a quick and satisfying breakfast or as a tasty snack.

Avocado Toast with Egg

Ingredients:

• 2 slices of whole-grain bread (or your choice of bread)

• 1 ripe avocado

• 2 large eggs

• Salt and black pepper to taste

• Optional toppings: red pepper flakes, hot sauce, sliced cherry tomatoes, feta cheese, or fresh herbs like cilantro or parsley

Instructions:

1. Place the slices of bread in a toaster or on a skillet over medium heat. Toast until they are golden brown and crisp.

2. While the bread is toasting, cut the ripe avocado in half. Remove the pit and scoop the flesh into a bowl. Mash the avocado with a fork until it reaches your desired level of creaminess. You can add a pinch of salt and black pepper to taste.

3. In a non-stick skillet, heat a bit of cooking oil or butter over medium heat. Crack the eggs into the skillet and cook them to your preferred style (sunny-side-up, over-easy, or scrambled).

4. If you're making sunny-side-up or over-easy eggs, cover the skillet with a lid briefly to help the eggs cook evenly and set the yolks without flipping them.

5. Sprinkle a pinch of salt and black pepper over the eggs for seasoning. Once the bread is toasted, spread the mashed avocado evenly over each slice.

6. Carefully transfer the cooked eggs onto the avocado-covered toast slices. If you like, you can add red pepper flakes, hot sauce, sliced cherry tomatoes, crumbled feta cheese, or fresh herbs for extra flavor and texture.

7. Your avocado toast with egg is ready to serve. Enjoy it as a delicious and wholesome breakfast or brunch.

Greek Yogurt and Berry Salad

Ingredients:

• 1 cup Greek yogurt (plain or flavored)

• 1 cup mixed berries (e.g., strawberries, blueberries, raspberries)

• 2 tablespoons honey or maple syrup (optional)

• 1/4 cup granola

• Fresh mint leaves for garnish (optional)

Instructions:

1. In a serving bowl, scoop out the Greek yogurt. Top the yogurt with mixed berries.

2. Drizzle honey or maple syrup over the berries for added sweetness if desired. Sprinkle granola on top for crunch and texture.

3. Garnish with fresh mint leaves for a burst of freshness.

Lentil and Spinach Salad

Ingredients:

- 1 cup cooked green lentils

- 2 cups fresh spinach leaves

- 1/4 cup diced red onion

- 1/4 cup crumbled feta cheese (optional)

- 2 tablespoons balsamic vinaigrette dressing

- Salt and pepper to taste

Instructions:

1. In a salad bowl, combine cooked green lentils, fresh spinach leaves, and diced red onion.

2. If desired, sprinkle crumbled feta cheese over the salad. Drizzle balsamic vinaigrette dressing over the salad.

3. Season with salt and pepper to taste. Toss the salad to combine all the ingredients.

Turkey and Vegetable Quinoa Bowl

Ingredients:

- 1 cup cooked quinoa

- 4 oz lean turkey breast, cooked and sliced

- 1 cup roasted vegetables (e.g., sweet potatoes, broccoli, cauliflower)

- 1/4 cup hummus

- 2 tablespoons tahini sauce

- Chopped fresh parsley for garnish (optional)

Instructions:

1. In a serving bowl, place cooked quinoa. Arrange slices of cooked turkey breast on top of the quinoa.

2. Add roasted vegetables to the bowl. Drizzle hummus and tahini sauce over the bowl.

3. Garnish with chopped fresh parsley if desired.

Quinoa and Spinach Stuffed Peppers

Ingredients:

• 4 bell peppers, any color

• 1 cup cooked quinoa

• 2 cups fresh spinach, chopped

• 1 cup canned black beans, drained and rinsed

• 1/2 cup diced tomatoes

• 1/2 cup shredded low-fat cheddar cheese

• 1 teaspoon cumin

• 1/2 teaspoon chili powder

• Salt and pepper to taste

• Olive oil for cooking

Instructions:

1. Preheat your oven to 375°F (190°C). Cut the tops off the bell peppers, remove seeds, and rinse them.

2. In a skillet, heat a bit of olive oil over medium heat. Add chopped spinach and cook until wilted.

3. In a large bowl, combine cooked quinoa, sautéed spinach, black beans, diced tomatoes, shredded cheddar cheese, cumin, chili powder, salt, and pepper.

4. Stuff each bell pepper with the quinoa mixture. Place the stuffed peppers in a baking dish and cover with aluminum foil.

5. Bake for about 30-35 minutes, or until the peppers are tender. Serve hot.

Grilled Chicken and Broccoli Salad

Ingredients:

• 2 boneless, skinless chicken breasts

• 4 cups broccoli florets

• 1/4 cup sliced almonds

• 1/4 cup dried cranberries

• 2 cups mixed greens

• 2 tablespoons balsamic vinaigrette dressing

• Olive oil for grilling

• Salt and pepper to taste

Instructions:

1. Preheat your grill to medium-high heat. Season chicken breasts with salt and pepper.

2. Grill the chicken for about 6-8 minutes per side, or until cooked through.

3. In a pot of boiling water, blanch the broccoli florets for 2-3 minutes, then drain and rinse with cold water. In a large salad bowl, combine mixed greens, blanched broccoli, sliced almonds, and dried cranberries.

4. Slice the grilled chicken and add it to the salad. Drizzle balsamic vinaigrette dressing over the salad and toss to combine.

5. Serve immediately.

Lentil and Vegetable Soup

Ingredients:

- 1 cup dried green or brown lentils, rinsed and drained

- 4 cups low-sodium vegetable broth

- 2 cups water

- 1 cup diced carrots

- 1 cup diced celery

- 1 cup diced onion

- 2 cloves garlic, minced

- 1 teaspoon dried thyme

- 1/2 teaspoon paprika

- Salt and pepper to taste

- Olive oil for sautéing

Instructions:

1. In a large pot, heat a bit of olive oil over medium heat.

2. Add diced onions, carrots, and celery. Sauté for about 5 minutes, until softened. Add minced garlic, dried thyme, paprika, salt, and pepper. Sauté for an additional minute.

3. Stir in lentils, vegetable broth, and water. Bring to a boil. Reduce heat, cover, and simmer for about 20-25 minutes, until lentils are tender.

4. Serve hot.

Tuna and White Bean Salad

Ingredients:

• 2 cans (5 oz each) tuna in water, drained

• 1 can (15 oz) white beans (cannellini or navy beans), drained and rinsed

• 1/2 red onion, finely chopped

• 1/2 cup chopped fresh parsley

• Juice of 1 lemon

• 2 tablespoons olive oil

• Salt and pepper to taste

Instructions:

1. In a large bowl, combine drained tuna, white beans, chopped red onion, and chopped fresh parsley.

2. Drizzle olive oil and lemon juice over the salad. Season with salt and pepper.

3. Toss everything together until well combined.

4. Serve chilled.

Sweet Potato and Lentil Bowl

Ingredients:

• 2 cups cooked brown rice

• 2 cups roasted sweet potatoes, cubed

• 1 cup cooked green or brown lentils

• 1 cup steamed broccoli florets

• 1/4 cup chopped walnuts

• 2 tablespoons balsamic vinaigrette dressing

• Salt and pepper to taste

Instructions:

1. In a large bowl, layer cooked brown rice, roasted sweet potatoes, cooked lentils, and steamed broccoli florets.

2. Drizzle balsamic vinaigrette dressing over the bowl. Sprinkle chopped walnuts on top.

3. Season with salt and pepper. Toss gently to combine. Serve warm.

Avocado and Black Bean Salad

Ingredients:

• Ripe avocados

• Canned black beans (drained and rinsed)

• Corn kernels (fresh or frozen)

• Chopped red onions

• Chopped cilantro

- Lime juice

- Olive oil

Instructions:

1. In a bowl, combine ripe avocados, black beans, corn kernels, chopped red onions, and chopped cilantro.

2. Drizzle with lime juice and olive oil, and gently toss to combine.

Baked Sweet Potato with Chickpea and Spinach Topping

Ingredients:

- Sweet potatoes

- Canned chickpeas (drained and rinsed)

- Chopped spinach

- Chopped red onion

- Olive oil

- Paprika

- Cumin

Instructions:

1. Preheat the oven to 400°F (200°C).

2. Pierce sweet potatoes with a fork and bake until tender.

3. In a pan, sauté chopped red onion, canned chickpeas, chopped spinach, olive oil, paprika, and cumin until spinach is wilted.

4. Split the baked sweet potatoes and top with the chickpea and spinach mixture.

Turkey and Avocado Wrap

Ingredients:

- Whole-grain wrap or tortilla

- Sliced turkey breast

- Sliced avocado

- Baby spinach leaves

- Dijon mustard (optional)

Instructions:

1. Lay a whole-grain wrap or tortilla flat.

2. Layer with sliced turkey breast, sliced avocado, baby spinach leaves, and a drizzle of Dijon mustard if desired.

3. Roll up the wrap and cut in half.

Sesame Kale and Tofu Salad

Ingredients:

• Chopped kale

• Baked or pan-fried tofu cubes

• Sliced cucumber

• Shredded carrots

• Sesame seeds

Sesame Ginger Dressing:

• Rice vinegar

• Sesame oil

- Soy sauce (low-sodium)

- Fresh ginger (grated)

- Honey

Instructions:

1. In a large bowl, combine chopped kale, baked or pan-fried tofu cubes, sliced cucumber, and shredded carrots.

2. In a separate bowl, whisk together the sesame ginger dressing ingredients.

3. Drizzle the dressing over the salad, sprinkle with sesame seeds, and toss to combine.

Mediterranean Lentil Soup

Ingredients:

- Green or brown lentils

- Chopped onions

- Chopped carrots

- Chopped celery

- Minced garlic

- Vegetable broth (low-sodium)

- Chopped tomatoes

- Ground cumin

- Paprika

- Fresh parsley (chopped)

Instructions:

1. In a large pot, combine green or brown lentils, chopped onions, chopped carrots, chopped celery, minced garlic, vegetable broth, chopped tomatoes, ground cumin, and paprika.

2. Simmer until lentils and vegetables are tender.

3. Serve garnished with fresh parsley.

Mushroom and Spinach Quinoa Bowl

Ingredients:

- Cooked quinoa

- Sautéed mushrooms

- Sautéed spinach

- Chopped roasted red peppers

- Feta cheese (optional)

Instructions:

1. Layer cooked quinoa, sautéed mushrooms, sautéed spinach, and chopped roasted red peppers in a bowl.

2. Sprinkle with feta cheese if desired.

Black Bean and Vegetable Quesadilla

Ingredients:

- Whole-grain tortilla

- Black beans (canned, rinsed, and mashed)

- Sliced bell peppers

- Sliced red onions

- Shredded low-fat cheese

- Salsa (optional)

Instructions:

1. Spread mashed black beans on a whole-grain tortilla.

2. Top with sliced bell peppers, sliced red onions, and shredded low-fat cheese.

3. Fold in half and cook on a skillet until cheese is melted.

4. Serve with salsa if desired.

Chickpea and Avocado Salad

Ingredients:

- Canned chickpeas (drained and rinsed)

- Diced avocado

- Chopped cucumber

- Chopped red onion

- Chopped cilantro

- Lime juice

• Olive oil

Instructions:

1. In a bowl, combine canned chickpeas, diced avocado, chopped cucumber, chopped red onion, and chopped cilantro.

2. Drizzle with lime juice and olive oil, and gently toss to combine.

Lentil and Spinach Stuffed Bell Peppers

Ingredients:

• Bell peppers (any color)

• Cooked green or brown lentils

• Sautéed spinach

• Chopped tomatoes

• Shredded low-fat cheese

Instructions:

1. Cut the tops off bell peppers and remove seeds and membranes.

2. Stuff the peppers with cooked lentils, sautéed spinach, chopped tomatoes, and shredded low-fat cheese.

3. Place the stuffed peppers in a baking dish and bake until peppers are tender.

Chicken and Quinoa Soup

Ingredients:

• Cooked chicken breast (shredded)

• Cooked quinoa

• Chopped carrots

• Chopped celery

• Chopped onions

• Low-sodium chicken broth

• Fresh thyme leaves

Instructions:

1. In a pot, combine shredded cooked chicken breast, cooked quinoa, chopped carrots, chopped celery, chopped onions, low-sodium chicken broth, and fresh thyme leaves.

2. Simmer until vegetables are tender.

Egg and Veggie Wrap

Ingredients:

• Whole-grain wrap or tortilla

• Scrambled eggs

• Sliced tomatoes

• Sliced bell peppers

• Sliced avocado

Instructions:

1. Lay a whole-grain wrap or tortilla flat.

2. Fill with scrambled eggs, sliced tomatoes, sliced bell peppers, and sliced avocado.

3. Roll up the wrap and enjoy.

Tuna and Quinoa Salad

Ingredients:

- Canned tuna (in water, drained)

- Cooked quinoa

- Sliced cucumbers

- Cherry tomatoes (halved)

- Kalamata olives (pitted and sliced)

- Greek dressing (olive oil, lemon juice, oregano)

Instructions:

1. In a bowl, combine canned tuna, cooked quinoa, sliced cucumbers, cherry tomatoes, and Kalamata olives.

2. Drizzle with Greek dressing and toss to combine.

Veggie and Hummus Wrap

Ingredients:

- Whole-grain wrap or tortilla

- Hummus

- Sliced cucumbers

- Sliced bell peppers

- Sliced red onions

- Baby spinach leaves

Instructions:

1. Lay a whole-grain wrap or tortilla flat.

2. Spread hummus over the wrap and layer with sliced cucumbers, sliced bell peppers, sliced red onions, and baby spinach leaves.

• 3. Roll up the wrap and enjoy.

Tomato and Basil Quinoa Salad

Ingredients:

• Cooked quinoa

• Chopped tomatoes

• Fresh basil leaves

• Balsamic vinaigrette (balsamic vinegar, olive oil, Dijon mustard)

Instructions:

1. In a bowl, combine cooked quinoa, chopped tomatoes, and fresh basil leaves.

2. Drizzle with balsamic vinaigrette and toss to combine.

Turkey and Cranberry Wrap

Ingredients:

• Whole-grain wrap or tortilla

• Sliced turkey breast

- Fresh spinach leaves

- Cranberry sauce (low-sugar)

- Chopped pecans

Instructions:

1. Lay a whole-grain wrap or tortilla flat.

2. Layer with sliced turkey breast, fresh spinach leaves, cranberry sauce, and chopped pecans.

3. Roll up the wrap and enjoy.

Salmon and Quinoa Stuffed Peppers

Ingredients:

- Bell peppers (any color)

- Baked or grilled salmon

- Cooked quinoa

- Chopped spinach

- Chopped tomatoes

- Olive oil

- Lemon juice

Instructions:

1. Cut the tops off bell peppers and remove seeds and membranes.

2. Fill the peppers with a mixture of baked or grilled salmon, cooked quinoa, chopped spinach, and chopped tomatoes.

3. Drizzle with olive oil and lemon juice.

4. Bake until the peppers are tender.

Vegetable and Chickpea Curry

Ingredients:

- Canned chickpeas (drained and rinsed)

- Mixed vegetables (e.g., cauliflower, carrots, peas)

- Chopped onions

- Coconut milk

- Curry powder

- Garlic and ginger (minced)

- Olive oil

Instructions:

1. In a large pan, sauté minced garlic and minced ginger in olive oil until fragrant.

2. Add chopped onions and mixed vegetables. Cook until softened.

3. Stir in canned chickpeas, coconut milk, and curry powder.

4. Simmer until the vegetables are tender.

Baked Sweet Potato and Black Bean Quesadillas

Ingredients:

- Whole-grain tortillas

- Mashed sweet potatoes

- Canned black beans (drained and rinsed)

- Sliced bell peppers

- Sliced red onions

- Low-fat cheese (shredded)

Instructions:

1. Lay out whole-grain tortillas.

2. Spread mashed sweet potatoes on half of each tortilla.

3. Top with black beans, sliced bell peppers, sliced red onions, and shredded low-fat cheese.

4. Fold the tortillas in half and cook on a skillet until golden brown.

Mushroom and Spinach Risotto

Ingredients:

- Arborio rice

- Sliced mushrooms

- Chopped spinach

- Chopped onions

- Low-sodium vegetable broth

- White wine (optional)

- Parmesan cheese (grated)

Instructions:

1. In a large skillet, sauté chopped onions and sliced mushrooms until soft.

2. Add Arborio rice and cook for a few minutes.

3. Pour in white wine (if using) and cook until it's mostly absorbed.

4. Gradually add low-sodium vegetable broth, stirring constantly until the rice is creamy.

5. Stir in chopped spinach and grated Parmesan cheese.

Turkey and Veggie Stir-Fry with Brown Rice

Ingredients:

- Ground turkey

- Sliced bell peppers

- Sliced carrots

- Sliced snow peas

- Low-sodium stir-fry sauce

- Garlic and ginger (minced)

- Brown rice

Instructions:

1. In a wok or skillet, cook ground turkey until browned.

2. Add sliced bell peppers, sliced carrots, and sliced snow peas. Stir-fry until the vegetables are tender.

3. Drizzle with low-sodium stir-fry sauce and serve over cooked brown rice.

Chickpea and Spinach Curry

Ingredients:

- Canned chickpeas (drained and rinsed)

- Chopped spinach

- Chopped onions

- Chopped tomatoes

- Coconut milk

- Curry powder

- Garlic and ginger (minced)

- Olive oil

Instructions:

1. In a large pan, sauté chopped onions, minced garlic, and minced ginger in olive oil until fragrant.

2. Add chopped tomatoes and cook until softened.

3. Stir in canned chickpeas, chopped spinach, coconut milk, and curry powder.

4. Simmer until spinach is wilted and the curry is heated through.

Baked Chicken and Broccoli Casserole

Ingredients:

• Boneless, skinless chicken breasts

• Steamed broccoli florets

• Brown rice

• Low-sodium chicken broth

• Shredded low-fat cheese

• Garlic powder

Instructions:

1. Preheat the oven to 375°F (190°C).

2. In a baking dish, layer cooked brown rice, steamed broccoli florets, and boneless, skinless chicken breasts.

3. Sprinkle with garlic powder and pour low-sodium chicken broth over the casserole.

4. Top with shredded low-fat cheese and bake until the chicken is cooked through.

Spinach and Salmon Salad

Ingredients:

- 4 cups fresh spinach leaves

- 1 grilled or baked salmon fillet (4-6 oz), flaked

- 1/4 cup cherry tomatoes, halved

- 1/4 cup sliced cucumbers

- 1/4 cup sliced red onions

- 1 tablespoon olive oil

- 1 tablespoon balsamic vinegar

- Salt and pepper to taste

Instructions:

1. In a large salad bowl, combine fresh spinach leaves, cherry tomatoes, sliced cucumbers, and sliced red onions.

2. Top the salad with the flaked salmon.

3. In a small bowl, whisk together olive oil, balsamic vinegar, salt, and pepper to create the dressing.

4. Drizzle the dressing over the salad, toss gently to coat, and serve.

Greek Chickpea Salad

Ingredients:

• 2 cups cooked chickpeas (canned or cooked from dried)

• 1 cup diced cucumbers

• 1 cup diced tomatoes

• 1/2 cup chopped red onions

• 1/2 cup crumbled feta cheese

• 1/4 cup chopped fresh parsley

• 2 tablespoons olive oil

• 2 tablespoons lemon juice

• Salt and pepper to taste

Instructions:

1. In a large salad bowl, combine cooked chickpeas, diced cucumbers, diced tomatoes, chopped red onions, crumbled feta cheese, and chopped fresh parsley.

2. In a small bowl, whisk together olive oil, lemon juice, salt, and pepper to make the dressing.

3. Drizzle the dressing over the salad, toss gently to combine, and serve.

Turkey and Avocado Wrap

Ingredients:

• Whole-grain wrap or tortilla

• 4 oz sliced turkey breast

• 1/4 avocado, sliced

• 1/2 cup mixed greens

• 1/4 cup sliced red bell pepper

• 1 tablespoon hummus (optional)

• Olive oil for cooking

Instructions:

1. Lay out the whole-grain wrap or tortilla. Spread a thin layer of hummus (if using) over the wrap.

2. Arrange sliced turkey breast, avocado slices, mixed greens, and sliced red bell pepper on the wrap. Roll up the wrap tightly, tucking in the sides as you go.

3. Slice in half diagonally for easier eating.

Broccoli and Quinoa Salad

Ingredients:

• 2 cups cooked quinoa

• 2 cups steamed broccoli florets

• 1/2 cup diced red bell pepper

• 1/2 cup diced red onion

• 1/4 cup sliced almonds

• 1/4 cup dried cranberries

- 2 tablespoons olive oil

- 2 tablespoons balsamic vinegar

- Salt and pepper to taste

Instructions:

1. In a large bowl, combine cooked quinoa, steamed broccoli florets, diced red bell pepper, diced red onion, sliced almonds, and dried cranberries.

2. In a small bowl, whisk together olive oil, balsamic vinegar, salt, and pepper to make the dressing.

3. Drizzle the dressing over the salad, toss gently to combine, and serve.

Tomato Basil Quinoa Bowl

Ingredients:

- 1 cup cooked quinoa

- 1 cup diced fresh tomatoes

- 1/4 cup chopped fresh basil

- 2 tablespoons grated Parmesan cheese

- 1 tablespoon olive oil

- 1 tablespoon balsamic vinegar

- Salt and pepper to taste

Instructions:

1. In a serving bowl, layer cooked quinoa, diced fresh tomatoes, and chopped fresh basil. Sprinkle grated Parmesan cheese on top.

2. In a small bowl, whisk together olive oil, balsamic vinegar, salt, and pepper to make the dressing.

3. Drizzle the dressing over the quinoa bowl and serve.

Baked Salmon with Lemon and Dill

Ingredients:

- 4 salmon fillets

- 2 lemons, thinly sliced

- 4 sprigs fresh dill

- 2 cloves garlic, minced

- 2 tablespoons olive oil

- Salt and pepper to taste

Instructions:

1. Preheat your oven to 375°F (190°C).

2. Place each salmon fillet on a separate piece of aluminum foil. Season the salmon with minced garlic, olive oil, salt, and pepper.

3. Top each fillet with lemon slices and a sprig of fresh dill. Seal the aluminum foil packets tightly.

4. Bake in the preheated oven for about 15-20 minutes, or until the salmon is cooked through and flakes easily with a fork.

5. Serve hot.

Quinoa and Black Bean Stuffed Peppers

Ingredients:

- 4 bell peppers, any color

- 1 cup cooked quinoa

- 1 cup canned black beans, drained and rinsed

- 1 cup diced tomatoes

- 1/2 cup corn kernels (fresh, frozen, or canned)

- 1/2 cup shredded cheddar cheese

- 1 teaspoon chili powder

- 1/2 teaspoon cumin

- Salt and pepper to taste

- Olive oil for cooking

Instructions:

1. Preheat your oven to 375°F (190°C). Cut the tops off the bell peppers, remove seeds, and rinse them.

2. In a skillet, heat a bit of olive oil over medium heat. Add diced tomatoes and corn kernels. Sauté for about 3-4 minutes until heated through.

3. In a large bowl, combine cooked quinoa, black beans, sautéed tomatoes and corn, shredded cheddar cheese, chili powder, cumin, salt, and pepper.

4. Stuff each bell pepper with the quinoa mixture. Place the stuffed peppers in a baking dish and cover with aluminum foil.

5. Bake for about 30-35 minutes, or until the peppers are tender.

6. Serve hot.

Chicken and Vegetable Stir-Fry

Ingredients:

• 2 boneless, skinless chicken breasts, cut into strips

• 2 cups broccoli florets

• 1 cup sliced bell peppers (assorted colors)

• 1 cup sliced carrots

• 1/2 cup sliced mushrooms

• 2 cloves garlic, minced

• 1/4 cup low-sodium soy sauce

- 2 tablespoons hoisin sauce

- 1 tablespoon sesame oil

- 2 tablespoons olive oil

- Cooked brown rice for serving

Instructions:

1. In a bowl, mix together low-sodium soy sauce, hoisin sauce, and sesame oil. Set aside.

2. In a large skillet or wok, heat olive oil over medium-high heat. Add minced garlic and sauté for about 30 seconds until fragrant.

3. Add chicken strips and stir-fry until they are no longer pink, about 5-6 minutes. Remove from the skillet and set aside.

4. In the same skillet, add a bit more olive oil if needed. Add broccoli florets, sliced bell peppers, sliced carrots, and sliced mushrooms. Stir-fry for about 5 minutes until the vegetables are tender-crisp.

5. Return the cooked chicken to the skillet. Pour the sauce mixture over the chicken and vegetables.

6. Stir-fry for an additional 2-3 minutes until everything is heated through. Serve the chicken and vegetable stir-fry over cooked brown rice.

Lentil and Sweet Potato Soup

Ingredients:

• 1 cup dried green or brown lentils, rinsed and drained

• 2 sweet potatoes, peeled and diced

• 1 onion, chopped

• 2 cloves garlic, minced

• 1 teaspoon ground cumin

• 1/2 teaspoon ground coriander

• 1/4 teaspoon ground turmeric

• 1/4 teaspoon smoked paprika

• 6 cups low-sodium vegetable broth

- 2 tablespoons olive oil

- Salt and pepper to taste

Instructions:

1. In a large pot, heat olive oil over medium heat.

2. Add chopped onions and minced garlic. Sauté for about 3-4 minutes until softened. Add diced sweet potatoes and cook for another 3-4 minutes.

3. Stir in ground cumin, ground coriander, ground turmeric, smoked paprika, salt, and pepper. Cook for an additional minute until fragrant.

4. Add rinsed lentils and vegetable broth to the pot.

5. Bring the mixture to a boil, then reduce heat, cover, and simmer for about 20-25 minutes, or until lentils and sweet potatoes are tender.

6. Serve hot.

Quinoa and Kale Salad with Citrus Vinaigrette

Ingredients:

- Cooked quinoa

- Chopped kale

- Sliced oranges or grapefruit

- Chopped almonds

- Feta cheese (optional)

Citrus Vinaigrette:

- Orange or grapefruit juice

- Olive oil

- Dijon mustard

- Honey

Instructions:

1. In a large bowl, combine cooked quinoa, chopped kale, sliced citrus fruit, and chopped almonds.

2. In a separate bowl, whisk together the citrus vinaigrette ingredients.

3. Drizzle the vinaigrette over the salad and toss to coat. Add feta cheese if desired.

Greek Salad with Grilled Shrimp

Ingredients:

• 1-pound large shrimp, peeled and deveined

• 4 cups mixed greens

• 1 cup cherry tomatoes, halved

• 1 cucumber, sliced

• 1/2 cup Kalamata olives, pitted and sliced

• 1/2 cup crumbled feta cheese

• 2 tablespoons olive oil

• 2 tablespoons lemon juice

• 1 teaspoon dried oregano

• Salt and pepper to taste

Instructions:

1. In a bowl, whisk together olive oil, lemon juice, dried oregano, salt, and pepper to make the dressing. Set aside.

2. Season the shrimp with a little olive oil, salt, and pepper. Grill the shrimp for about 2-3 minutes per side, or until they turn pink and opaque.

3. In a large salad bowl, combine mixed greens, cherry tomatoes, cucumber slices, Kalamata olives, and crumbled feta cheese.

4. Add the grilled shrimp on top of the salad.

5. Drizzle the dressing over the salad, toss gently to coat, and serve.

CONCLUSION

Osteoporosis is a common and often silent disease that can lead to severe consequences if left untreated. It weakens bones, making them fragile and prone to fractures, particularly in the hip, spine, and wrist. However, osteoporosis is not an inevitable part of aging, and there are effective strategies for prevention and management.

Exercise is a cornerstone of osteoporosis management, offering a multitude of benefits for individuals affected by this condition. Exercise plays a pivotal role in the prevention and management of osteoporosis. Weight-bearing exercises, strength training, balance and posture exercises, flexibility routines, low-impact aerobics activities, and breathing exercises all contribute to better bone health and overall well-being.

Regular exercise offers several advantages for individuals with osteoporosis, including improved bone density, strengthened muscles, enhanced balance and coordination, a reduced risk of falls, increased joint mobility, and cardiovascular benefits. It is essential to consult with a healthcare provider or physical therapist before starting an exercise program, especially for those with osteoporosis. Exercises should be tailored to an individual's specific condition, age, and fitness level to ensure safety and effectiveness.

Osteoporosis is a serious condition that requires attention, but it is not without effective solutions. Exercise, when incorporated as part of a comprehensive management strategy, can significantly improve bone health, reduce the risk of fractures, enhance overall physical function, and contribute to a higher quality of life. By taking proactive steps, including exercise, individuals with osteoporosis can continue to lead active, fulfilling lives while minimizing the impact of this condition on their well-being.

www.ingramcontent.com/pod-product-compliance
Lightning Source LLC
Chambersburg PA
CBHW072215290526
45794CB00004B/1759